The Dukan Diet

*A High Protein Diet Plan To Help You Lose Weight
And Keep It Off For Life*

By Susan T. Williams

Table of Contents

Introduction

Thank you very much for downloading *'The Dukan Diet — A High Protein Diet Plan To Help You Lose Weight And Keep It Off For Life'*.

The Dukan Diet was created by French nutritionist and doctor, Pierre Dukan. It all started back in 1975 when he was approached by a client who was suffering from obesity. This client wanted to know if there was a way he could lose weight while still eating a lot of meat. This caused Dukan to take a step back from his normal way of thinking and consider an alternative to dieting. At that stage, it was a simple case of cutting back on calories and eating smaller meals and changing this would be difficult and certainly talked about. He had to be smart about it and make sure he did his research. Twenty years later he published his findings in a book titled 'Je ne sais pas maigrir', translated in English as 'I don't know how to lose weight'. It immediately became a bestseller.

The diet shows people how to lose weight and keep it off without spending hours at the gym. The clever title behind his strategy was 'The real reason the French stay thin'. It became so popular that even Kate Middleton and her mother decided to give it a try. The aim was to lose a bit of weight before the big wedding to Prince William and look good in her dress. It worked, she lost the weight, looked brilliant, and soon the whole world wanted to know what this diet was all about.

The Dukan Diet is implemented in four stages:

The Attack Phase
The Cruise Phase
The Consolidation Phase
The Stabilization Phase

In this book we take a closer look at the diet, through all four stages, and we will see how you can take this diet and make it work for you.

CHAPTER 1

The Skinny on the Dukan Diet

What makes the Dukan Diet so popular is that it has been devised into clear and definable phases, making the process easier and more manageable. Too many times people just throw themselves into a weight loss regime and then fail because they become too overwhelmed by everything they can and cannot do. Without clear guidelines it becomes impossible to succeed. In this diet, Pierre Dukan created a four point phase system. In the first two stages it is all about losing the weight, so results are quick and efficient. The next two stages focus more on maintaining and stabilizing your weight once you have reached this True Weight. So by the end it becomes more of a lifestyle than a diet, making it easier to manage on a day-to-day basis.

By including different phases into the diet, it becomes a lot easier to follow. We aren't just thrown into a whole new eating plan and then left to our own devices. Instead, Pierre Dukan has carefully put together a well thought out plan that allows us to move at our own pace throughout each phase. This is a very personal journey, and through these phases we can work towards a goal that suits us individually.

Your 'True Weight' is the weight you are trying to achieve, and one that is both realistic and healthy in terms of your body and its needs. In a recent ad, various women's bodies were shown at 130 lbs (60 kg), and each one looked completely different from the next. That is why weight should be based on your unique body and nobody else. Bone structure, height, family history, age and gender all play a role in what your True Weight should be. So before you start, make sure you have a realistic goal in mind.

The Dukan Diet was not something that was devised overnight. Instead it took years of research to reach where it is today. It's interesting to note that while the first two phases were developed in 1975, the second two phases were added five years later. To this day, Pierre Dukan continues to work methodically, making sure that each element of the diet is perfect.

What's the skinny on exercise?

Before we delve into the four stages of the diet, let's take a quick look at how much exercise you need to do to get great results from this diet.

While exercise is vital to this plan, it is important to note that this doesn't mean you have to exercise for hours at a time each day. Dukan believes that the most important thing about exercise is incorporating the art of movement into your daily life and learning how to make the right choices each time. Low impact exercises will keep you fit and healthy without causing injury. For the most, it's about having fun and allowing exercise to become something that you enjoy rather than dread. After all, if you are not enjoying it, then it simply won't become part of your daily habits and routines. You'll do it for a while and then stop. If you want to create positive and long lasting changes, then you have to make sure you are doing things that are feasible in the long term.

Pierre Dukan has devised a six point easy exercise plan to help you get started:

Don't take the elevator, take the stairs instead. We're all guilty of taking the elevator when given the option, because even very fit people find the stairs quite daunting. But stairs are a fantastic way of adding movement into your life, giving you a cardiovascular workout that's both good for the heart as well as the body. Best of all, it's proven to be one of the best ways to get a firm butt. So next time you see stairs, think of this and get going. The more stairs you have to climb, the better.

Walk your dog. Kill two birds with one stone here by not only making your dog happy but losing weight at the same time. It's a good way to be out of the house enjoying the fresh air. It allows you time for self-reflection.

Use your lunch breaks wisely. What do you do in your lunch hour? Sit at your desk? Sit in the kitchen area? The truth is that most jobs these days require a lot of sitting, so if you have any opportunity to break from this, you should do so. Get out and stretch your legs. It's a great way of getting in some much needed movement into your day.

Dance like nobody is watching. Dancing is one of the best ways to lose weight and tone, and what's better is that you'll have fun doing it! It's also a great way to learn a new hobby to incorporate into your life. Learning new dance moves is good for the body, mind and soul. Sign up for that salsa class you've been eyeing, or think about taking that Zumba class at your local gym. But if you have two left feet, and the thought of dancing in a group scares you, then just dance at home. Put on some music and dance to your own rhythm. *Just Dance* for the Nintendo Wii is a great way to dance at home and get some needed exercise. Again, it's all about movement and having fun.

Shop until you drop. The best part about retail therapy is that you're getting in quite a lot of walking without realizing it. Through all the distractions it won't even feel like exercising, but you'll get a whole lot more fitter walking around the mall than sitting on the couch at home. Plus, you'll walk away with some brand new clothes.

Mow the lawn. Starting and maintaining a garden is a fantastic way to keep fit. A garden is a lot of work and a great way to work up a sweat. The best part is that you are not only working towards a better looking garden, but also a better looking you.

CHAPTER 2

The Attack Phase

T his is the first phase of the four step process. It's an exciting time because it means you have finally decided to take the first step towards a healthier lifestyle. Due to this sudden change in diet, your body will react and you'll probably lose the most weight. This phase is also known as the Pure Protein phase.

So how long does this phase last?

The duration of the Attack Phase depends entirely on you. As a guideline, Dukan suggests the following:

To lose under 10 pounds – stay in this phase for 1 – 2 days.

To lose between 15 – 30 pounds – stay in this phase for 3 – 5 days.

To lose more than 40 pounds – stay in this phase for up to 7 days (but consult with your physician before starting).

What does this phase entail?

In this phase you can eat as much as you want as long as it is on the allowed foods list. The aim is to introduce you to a different way of eating by making sure you adhere to strict rules and guidelines. There are three very important things you need to keep in mind while in the Attack Phase.

Firstly you need to make sure you are properly hydrated with water. Allow yourself to drink 1.5 liters or more per day. This may seem difficult for many people who are not used to drinking water, so the best advice I can give is to fill a bottle with water and put it on your desk next to you. Actually seeing the water will remind you that you need to drink it, and eventually it will become a habit. Another option is to set a reminder on your phone every half an hour or hour to have water. This is an incredibly important part of the process and must not be eliminated.

Secondly, you must incorporate a twenty minute walk (or similar) every single day. Of course if you are already a very fit person than you can continue to exercise as you are used to. For those new to exercise, it is important that you get in at least twenty minutes of gentle exercise.

Lastly, the final thing that is part of the diet and important, especially in this phase, is to include 1.5 tablespoons of oat bran into each day. While this is easy for a lot of people, many are not sure how to incorporate this in a way that is pleasing to them. So Pierre Dukan devised a recipe that has become a staple for many people, called The Oat Bran Galette. It can be made in bulk and stored in the fridge to use daily. Here is the recipe for two servings.

Ingredients:

2 whole eggs
3 tablespoons of oat bran (this will change if you are in another phase so bare that in mind. Also remember this serves two, which is why it has 3 tablespoons. This will be 4 tablespoons in the Cruise Phase)
3 tablespoons of 0% fat Greek yogurt (4 tablespoons in the Cruise Phase)

Method:

1. Whisk all the ingredients together until you have a smooth liquid batter.
2. Grease the bottom of a non-stick pan.
3. Spoon half the mixture in and cook the pancake on medium heat until golden brown on both sides.
4. Repeat this process for the second pancake.

What foods are allowed?

The most important thing in this phase is to stick to the foods allocated and to keep all foods to fewer than 5% fat, unless otherwise stated. Those that stick to this food guideline without any deviation are those that see the best results.

The foods that you can eat during this phase are:
Low-fat dairy products (skimmed milk is fine, avoid fruit flavored yogurt)
Chicken (without the skin)
Turkey (without the skin)
Lean beef (under 10% fat)
Veal
Rabbit
Beef
Chicken liver
Fish (unless it is canned in oil or sauce)
Shellfish
Eggs (two a day of whole eggs, and unlimited egg whites)
Sweeteners (unless they are fructose based)

Spices, herbs, vinegar, lemon juice
Coffee and tea (without sugar)

While drinking water is the most important part of this phase and this diet as a whole, it is almost important to realize that there are other drinks allowed. This might be helpful for those moments when you are feeling hunger pangs in this first phase. With regards to water you can have still or sparkling (add a few drops of lemon juice to add flavor). Tea and coffee is also allowed as long as it has skimmed milk and no sugar (low calorie sweeteners are allowed if desired). Sugar free drinks such as Coke Zero and Diet Pepsi are also allowed.

To get you started, here are some ideas for a full day of food:

Day one:
Breakfast: Scrambled eggs with bacon and a cup of coffee
Snack: Low-fat yogurt
Lunch: Oat bran galette with cream cheese and turkey, and a cup of tea.
Dinner: Spicy lemon roast chicken (see recipe section in the last chapter)

Day two:
Breakfast: Grilled chicken with low fat cottage cheese and a cup of coffee
Snack: Oat bran muffins and a cup of tea
Lunch: Omelet with cheese and ham
Dinner: Turkey meatballs (see recipe section in the last chapter)

How will I feel?

One of the biggest questions people ask before embarking on the Dukan Diet is: *how will I feel?* It's important to note that phase one is going to be a complete shock to the system. Although a pure protein phase might sound easy, the truth is that your body has probably gotten very used to including carbs and vegetables with each meal. Often, it becomes more a case of dealing with personal demons as you struggle to come to terms with not eating certain things. Without realizing it you have more than likely become quite addicted to carbs or chocolate and taking it away completely will not only have an effect on your body but also your mind. You need to fight through the first few days because it *will* get easier.

A great idea is to make sure your kitchen is fully stocked with all the foods on the allowed list and to rid it of anything that is not. You want to make sure you have little to no temptation throughout this stage.

You might also feel tired for the first few days, but don't worry as that is a completely normal feeling as your body is adjusting to this new way of eating. Soon enough you'll feel better. In fact, you'll probably feel more energized than you have in a very long time.

Never skip meals, have yogurt if you start to crave sugar, drink coffee and tea in between meals, and drink plenty of water. Mostly, stay positive and be kind to yourself in this time.

How often should I weigh myself?

As your body is adjusting to this huge change in diet, you should start to see a big change in the scale as your weight goes down. This is the stage in which people lose weight the fastest (although not everyone is the same, so please don't be discouraged if you don't see a huge difference here). During this stage it is important to monitor your weight regularly as it will help you determine when you are ready to go onto the next phase, and will also help to boost your morale during this hard period.

Bear in mind, though, that many factors contribute towards the number on the scale so don't get too caught up in the numbers and try focus more on how your body feels and how your clothes feel. If you weigh yourself, try stick to the same routine each time. By this I mean weigh yourself at the same time every day, preferably first thing in the morning before your body gets heavy during the day. Weigh yourself in the same place and wear the same clothes. If you move your scale from one room to another it might change the number due to how level the ground is or whether you you've gone from tiles to carpet. So be consistent in the weighing process.

Other factors come into play such as whether you've exercised, what you've eaten, how much water you've had, whether or not you are on your period, etc. So at the end of the day, use the numbers as a guideline but nothing more. If you're the type of person to become easily obsessed about whether the numbers drop, then it is okay to skip this altogether. At the end of the day it is not about what the numbers say but about how you feel about yourself. You'll know if you've lost weight without a device telling you so.

CHAPTER 3

The Cruise Phase

During the second phase of the Dukan Diet you will start to reintroduce certain vegetables into your diet. Here you'll find your weight loss less rapid than it was in the first phase, but this slower and steadier phase will help you to eventually reach your True Weight. The most important part of this phase is to rid your body of all excess fat while still conserving a lean body mass.

The best part about this phase is the introduction of 32 non-starchy vegetables into your diet, which makes meal time recipes a lot easier to put together. You'll start to feel like this is more of a lifestyle than a diet which helps both the body and the mind, and you'll also start to have a lot more fun in the cooking process. At the end of the day you don't want to constantly be 'on a diet' so creating a lifestyle with healthy choices is what you are eventually trying to achieve. While phase one was an introduction into a new way of eating, phase two is a way of showing you how you can incorporate this into your everyday life. Through slow and positive changes you will eventually find this new way of eating easy and beneficial.

So how long does this phase last?

This phase will last as long as you need it to. In other words it all boils down to when you reach your goal weight because as soon as you do, you will move on to the third phase which is all about maintaining your weight. The more weight you need to lose the longer you will be required to stay in this stage. It is important not to become obsessed with a certain number, because while you may have had a number in mind, your True Weight might have changed in the process. In this instance it is vital that you consider how you feel and how you look in your clothes. Your new goal weight might be slightly less than you originally thought or it might also be slightly more. Often, we think we need to lose more than we really need. It's all about focusing on what makes you feel good.

What does this phase entail?

The Cruise Phase involves alternating your pure-protein days (PP) with protein and vegetable days (PV). While there is no strict rule on how you want to do this, most people have found that just doing one day PV and one day PP is the easiest to maintain and remember. Weight loss might be a little slower should you choose the PP / PV method, but it will be easier to remember when you should be eating what. However, this is completely up to you and your lifestyle. A lot of people like to do five pure protein days followed by five protein and vegetable days. This method, while effective, can be very hard to follow as it requires a lot more dedication and motivation. Another popular system is doing seven days pure protein and seven days protein and vegetables. While this is quite difficult for many people, a lot of people prefer this because they know exactly which days require them to do what type of eating. So if they start the program on a Monday with pure protein they know that the following Monday they'll be on protein and vegetables. Once again, it's up to you. The nice thing about this diet is that you can change it up slightly to fit your particular needs.

Including oat bran into this phase is just as important as it was in phase one. The only difference is that you are now going to be having 2 tablespoons of oat bran instead of 1.5. Remember this when you are making your oat bran galette.

Once again, exercise becomes a crucial part of this phase. While it was important to walk at least 20 minutes each day in the Attack Phase this will now change to 30 minutes or more in the Cruise Phase. Once again, if you are already quite a fit person, then feel free to push yourself harder with exercise.

What foods are allowed?

The foods allowed in this phase are a lot more varied. In total, there are 100 foods allowed in the Dukan Diet, and we'll take a closer look at that at the end of the book. Please be aware that a protein only diet causes your body to lose water quite rapidly which is why it is vital that you drink a lot of water in the process. As soon as you start introducing vegetables again, your body will naturally begin to retain the water. Remember that this is very normal, as your body is adjusting to the new routine.

The vegetables that you are now allowed to introduce into your diet are:

Artichoke	Kale
Asparagus	Lettuce
Bean sprouts	Mushrooms
Beetroot (in moderation, as they are	Onion
starchy)	Okra
Broccoli	Palm hearts
Brussels sprouts	Peppers
Cabbage	Pumpkin
Carrots (in moderation, as they are	Radish
starchy)	Rhubarb

Cauliflower	Spaghetti squash
Celery	Spinach
Cucumber	Squash
Eggplant	Tomatoes
Endive	Turnip
Fennel	Watercress
Green beans	Zucchini

It's important to note that foods such as potatoes, beans, peas, lentils and avocado are still banned. Print out a list of your allowed foods, make sure your fridge and cupboards are filled with only these items, and you'll be fine. While each person is different, the general rule is that it takes three days per pound you want to lose. While this is a rough estimate, you can at least get an idea of how long you will be on this phase for.

While there is no set portion control for each meal, the best and most efficient way to lose weight is to just eat until you feel sufficiently full and energized.

To get you started, here are some ideas for a full day of food:

Day one (PP):
Breakfast: Egg white omelet with ham, cheese and chives, and a cup of coffee
Snack: Low-fat yogurt and a cup of tea
Lunch: Oat bran galette with cream cheese and turkey, and a glass of diet Pepsi
Dinner: Ground meat stuffed peppers (see recipe section in the last chapter)

Day two (PV):
Breakfast: Scrambled eggs with asparagus and a cup of coffee
Snack: Carrot sticks dipped in low-fat cheese
Lunch: Oat bran galette with lettuce, tomato and bacon
Dinner: Chili con Dukan (see recipe section in the last chapter)

How will I feel?

It is not uncommon for people to put on a bit of weight as they enter this phase from the Attack Phase. Of course, after losing weight so rapidly in the first phase this can sometimes come as a bit of shock and many people feel scared or depressed. Please understand that this is natural, and you will lose that weight again quickly. This is just your body's way of dealing with the change in diet and adjusting to this sudden extra nourishment it is getting. As mentioned earlier, it is more than likely that your body is now just storing extra water, because in the Attack Phase your body got very used to losing water quickly. In the Cruise Phase, your body tries to rebalance itself by hanging onto the extra water it is getting through vegetables. This is all very normal, and soon your body will get back into a balanced state and will stop storing all the water that comes in. Continue with your diet, and continue drinking water during this period. If you are aware of these changes, you will find it easier to get through the first few days of this phase.

How often should I weigh myself?

It is definitely recommended that you weigh yourself less during the Cruise Phase, mostly because you will not be losing weight as quickly as you did in the previous phase, and you may feel despondent at the numbers. Your body will start resisting weight loss which can sometimes be quite a frustrating time to go through. This could be the result of two things. Firstly, it could just mean that you are fast approaching your goal weight, or that you might already be at your goal weight. It is during this time that you need to assess how much you have lost, how much you wanted to lose and how happy you are at this moment. Secondly, it could just mean that you need to change things up a little because your body might just be getting lazy and used to the process. An easy way of doing this would be to change up your system of pure protein days versus protein and vegetables days. So if you were going the one day PP / one day PV route then maybe try doing a five day PP / five day PV route. Also, you might need to start exercising more. You are probably just getting fitter and healthier, and your body might just need to be pushed a little more as far as exercise.

CHAPTER 4

The Consolidation Phase

This is the third phase of the Dukan Diet and certainly a very exciting and crucial phase to be in. It's exciting because it means that you have completed the first two phases of the diet, and you have now reached your goal weight. So before we go any further, this is now the time for you to take a step back and congratulate yourself. You've shown that you have the dedication and the determination to get the results you want and you should be proud of what you have accomplished. The mere fact that you have gotten so far means that the next two phases should be easy for you. This is the time to realize that this is not a diet but a way of life, and while phase one and two were just preparation for this lifestyle, the time has now come to maintain it. How wonderful to know that you are now in the third phase of the diet, with only one phase left. You've made it this far and you can definitely go all the way.

So how long does this phase last?

The length of the Consolidation Phase is dependent on how much weight you have lost in the first two phases. The general rule is that you need five days of phase three for every pound that you have lost. So if you have lost two pounds you need to be in this phase for ten days, and so on. By completing this stage, it will allow you to form positive habits to keep your weight off for good. This is a very important phase because it not uncommon for people to put weight back on after a diet and then slowly spiral out of control. By making sure you get through the whole of phase three, you will be ensuring that this doesn't happen.

What does this phase entail?

While still using what you have learnt from phase one and two, you will now be allowed to introduce a few more foods into your diet. This will make the process easier and more manageable as a lifestyle for you. However, so that you don't suddenly undo everything that you have learned, you have to follow some very strict guidelines when introducing the new foods into your eating schedule. We will go over that next. The Consolidation Phase is what makes this diet different from any other. It is through this phase that other foods are allowed back in, ensuring that this diet works for you in the long run. While many other diets suddenly just stop when you reach your goal weight, this one has been designed so that the weight stays off forever. If you stick with this phase, you will not regret doing so and you will be able to stay at your goal weight for the rest of your life. Admittedly this phase can be difficult for some because they feel almost as if they are not on 'diet' anymore and eat more than they should. However if you stick to the plan you will not fail!

What foods are allowed?

You are allowed everything that you had in phase one and two. By now you should be quite used to eating this way so this shouldn't be a problem. However, there are rules attached to the extra foods allowed in this phase:

Firstly you must divide your Consolidation Phase into two sections, the first half and the second half. You will know how many days your phase will last by how many pounds you have lost, so this should be easy to calculate.

First half of the Consolidation Phase:

You are now allowed one serving of fruit a day. However this does not include bananas, grapes, figs or cherries. Berries, strawberries and oranges are always great choices.

You can now introduce two pieces of whole grain bread a day.

1.5 ounces (40 grams) of hard rind cheese can now be introduced. This includes Gouda, Swiss cheese and cheddar. Avoid goat cheese, Camembert (brie) and Roquefort.

1 serving of starchy foods a week. Once a week, you can now include a serving (1 cup cooked) of starch to your meals, however try to avoid white rice and potatoes. Instead choose whole grain pasta, whole grain rice, lentils and beans.

And now for the best part-- the Dukan Diet now allows for 1 celebration meal a week. After all, this phase should be a celebration of what you have achieved. A celebration meal includes one appetizer, one entrée, one dessert and one glass of wine. Please be advised that you can only have one serving of each.

Second half of the Consolidation Phase:

You are now allowed two servings of fruit a day. Again this does not include bananas, grapes, figs or cherries.

You can still enjoy two pieces of whole grain bread a day.

1.5 ounces (40 grams) of hard rind cheese can still be eaten. Again, this includes Gouda, Swiss cheese and cheddar. Avoid goat cheese, Camembert (brie) and Roquefort.

You can now enjoy 2 servings of starchy foods a week. The same rules apply as before.

2 celebration meals can now be enjoyed a week.

To include in the entire Consolidation Phase:

You should always include one Protein Thursday (known as PP Thursday) into your week, where no vegetables or carbohydrates are consumed. It is imperative that you stick with this in order to maintain your True Weight. Of course this doesn't specifically have to be a Thursday; however it should be the same day each week to make it easier for you to remember. Most people have found Thursday to be the best day because they then enjoy the celebration meal on Friday. This makes Thursday a lot easier to deal with.

Exercise should still be a vital part of this phase. Make sure that you are doing at least 25 minutes of brisk walking a day or more.

Remember it is still important to include 2 tablespoons of oat bran a day, although by now you should be quite used to having this as part of your diet.

For all the meals in this phase, you should stick to a 225 g serving or less. White rice and potatoes are allowed, but it is advised to stick to brown rice. If you do choose white rice, then perhaps have a smaller serving. Also, if you do want potatoes, then always cook them in their skins.

How will I feel?

The Consolidation Phase is different for each person. Most people will enjoy the extra freedom and feel better now that they are allowed a bigger variety in their diet. Also, they will find their one day of pure protein to be easier than before because they know that the next day they will be able to enjoy something else. So for the most part, this phase is a good change from the one before, and certainly much better than the Attack Phase.

However, this is the stage in which some people fail. The introduction of new foods can set them into a downward spiral. Some people find being on a strict diet a lot easier to follow than the freedom that this phase allows. They are not able to stop themselves during the celebration meal and will go back for seconds, even though this is not allowed. In turn they will feel guilty and will often stop the program altogether.

It is important to be aware of what might happen, so that you can stop it when it does. And if you do cheat, don't let that be the end of your journey. Understand why you have done it and simply start again the next day. You don't have to start all the way from the beginning. You just have to carry on from where you left off. Mostly it's about being kind to yourself and understanding that you are only human. Laugh it off and keep going. Be strong during this time, and you will be fine.

CHAPTER 5

The Stabilization Phase

You're now on the fourth and final phase of the Dukan Diet. A huge accomplishment and one that should be celebrated with great pride and joy. You've gotten to your goal weight and you've done it through healthy and long lasting methods. By now you have set positive habits into your life that will never leave you. You've finally learned how to create a lifestyle for yourself that allows you to enjoy food while still eating for the health of both your body and mind. So congratulations! Take some time to really enjoy this moment.

This phase was created by Pierre Dukan in 1999 in his popular book 'Je ne c'est pas maigrir', after he saw the importance of not only losing the weight but keeping it off for good. What was the point of going through such a big diet with so many changes, if you were just going to rush back to normal afterwards and put it all back on? He saw what happens with other diets, how people end up putting the weight back on, but they end up putting on more than they had when they started out. That is when depression sets in and when bad food habits start to form.

The Stabilization Phase was designed to stop all that from happening.

So how long does this phase last?

As this is the final stage of the diet, this phase quite simply doesn't end. By now you have figured out how to incorporate this new way of eating and living into your life. This is now a lifestyle and not a diet. This phase is how you should remain from here onwards, and it's an exciting place to be. It means you have been through the highs and lows of phases one, two and three, and you have finally reached a point of balance. Remember all the lessons you learned from the previous phases and take them into your life as you continue with this new way of eating.

What does this phase entail?

Here there are a few rules that you need to adhere to so that you can continue to keep your weight off and feel healthy. These rules are only here to guide you now in order for you to continue on this positive path that you have been on.

Some of the rules are:

Continue with Protein Thursday (or whatever day you have chosen). This is a fantastic reminder of what you have been through and helps your body to have one day where it completely breaks off from any other foods that you have now introduced into your diet. This one day should involve no other foods but protein, just as you did in your Attack Phase. Sticking to one specific day a week will continue to assure that you follow this rule with ease.

Continue to eat your oat bran every day. This will aid in the digestion process and will reduce the amount of carbohydrates absorbed. It is a great way to keep all cravings at bay. Again, by now you should be so used to eating this that it shouldn't be a problem to continue with it. You can continue eating your oat bran galette, and now you can include more interesting foods in your diet. Most people continue to use the oat bran galette as a staple in their diet.

Exercise often. It is important that you continue to exercise each and every day. The amount you do is completely up to you, but make sure that you feel yourself getting a proper cardiovascular workout. For some this might just be a brisk half an hour walk daily, for others it might be more of a higher impact sport. Do whatever suits you and your lifestyle and just make sure that it is something you stick to every day. This is one of the key elements for losing weight and has other amazing benefits for both morale and the mind. Other than having a dedicated time to exercise every day, you should also always try to incorporate movement into your days by taking the stairs instead of the lift and walking instead of taking the car. They might seem like small changes, but they offer big rewards.

CHAPTER 6

Implementing the Dukan diet into your life

So let's do a quick recap on the four phases:

The Attack Phase - This is the first phase of the four steps, and it is used to jump start the weight loss process. It involves a protein-only diet with strict guidelines. You stay on this diet according to how much weight you need to lose in the first place. Due to this sudden change in diet it means this is where you'll probably lose the most weight.

The Cruise Phase - This is the second phase of the Dukan Diet where you will start to reintroduce certain vegetables into your diet. Here you'll find your weight loss less rapid than it was in the first phase, but this slower and steadier phase will help you to eventually reach your True Weight. The most important part of this phase is to rid your body of all excess fat while still conserving a lean body mass.

The Consolidation Phase - This is the third phase of the Dukan Diet and will help you to prevent a rebound from happening, and certainly a very exciting and crucial phase to be in. This is the time to realize that this is not a diet but a way of life, and while phase one and two were just preparation for this lifestyle, the time has now come to maintain it.

The Stabilization Phase - The fourth and final phase of the Dukan Diet. This is when the diet becomes part and parcel of your every life and you use the lessons that you learned from the first three phases in order to create a better lifestyle for yourself. This phase was created in order for this new way of living to become a part of your life forever.

The Nutritional Staircase:

Pierre Dukan has put together seven points which make up the nutritional staircase; these are in order of most important to least important.

Proteins. Most important. This is vital to your diet. This diet will teach you how to incorporate pure protein days into each week.

Vegetables. Essential. After the Attack Phase this becomes an important part to add to the diet.

Fruits. Important. While these should not be eaten as often as proteins and vegetables it is still good to include some of these into your diet each day.

Bread. Helpful. As long as you are not eating bread with each meal, it is still a good form of nutrition for the body.

Cheese. Nutrition and pleasure. Cheese is a fantastic addiction to most meals, however while it might taste good, too much is not a good thing. So just make sure you eat this sparingly.

Starches. Energy. Starchy food is great for energy; however they should not be eaten too often. More active people can enjoy starchy food as they need the energy.

Celebration meals. Pure pleasure. The least important of all the steps, however good for morale purposes and to allow you to still enjoy the foods you love in moderation.

Tips:

Be good to yourself. Remember where you were when you first started this process. It's often easy to lose yourself and forget why you wanted to change in the first place. Most people are too hard on themselves when it comes to losing weight and keeping it off and forget about how much they have already accomplished. Celebrate yourself through all four stages and be proud that you have taken the step towards a better life.

Remember the importance of balance. You're now not on a strict diet anymore, however this doesn't mean that you can go crazy. Listen to your body and allow yourself to stop eating when you are nourished and to also try to eat the right things where possible. Even diet drinks and sugar free gum should be consumed in smaller quantities. Don't reach for a second helping. Most of the time you do not need it. Instead, reach for a glass of water, and allow your body to feel full.

If you have something planned with friends or family, perhaps a night out at a restaurant, then make sure that this is your celebration meal for the week. This will allow you to have a guilt-free evening, knowing that the next day you will be back to a normal diet day.

Noticing some weight coming back on? Don't stress. Introduce two pure protein days into your week until you are back to your True Weight.

Learn how to cook without fat. The best way to do this is to use a steamer or a microwave for most of your meals. Also by using spices in the cooking process you'll find that you don't actually need the fat in order for your food to taste good. If you need to use the oven or the stove, then make sure you use non-stick pans and silicone molds for baking. Once again it is all about making the right choices in each meal and sometimes the smallest things can make a big difference.

Use Shirataki noodles instead of pasta. This is allowed on the Dukan Diet, and will make a great replacement for all those pasta dishes you are used to making.

Take the normal meals that you enjoy and find ways to turn them into a Dukan friendly meal. This might just mean swapping certain items for items that are allowed on the Dukan allowed foods list.

When using stock cubes (or bouillon cubes) make sure you go for a low fat or reduced salt version.

Desperately need a snack? Craving something sweet? Sugar free jelly is the way to go as long as it doesn't have any fruit included.

What are the benefits of Oat Bran?

Oat bran is an important part of the Dukan Diet due to its important nutritional value. Pierre Dukan has put together four reasons why you should be eating it daily:

It's delicious. It can be incorporated into your diet in so many different ways which makes it a wonderfully versatile product. It is a crucial part of the entire diet, in particular during the Attack Phase, because it is a great source of carbohydrates.

Lowers cholesterol. Oat bran reduces the bad cholesterol in the body by reducing the absorption into the bloodstream. Due to its high fiber content, it has a wonderfully soothing effect on the digestive system.

It keeps you feeling full. One of the best things about oat bran is that it keeps you feeling fuller for longer, which is exactly what you need when you are trying to lose weight. This means are less likely to reach for unnecessary snacks.

Slows down sugar and fat absorption. The process that the oat bran goes through in your body slows down the buildup of sugar and removes calories from the body.

The 100 foods that are allowed on this diet

There are 100 foods that are allowed on the Dukan Diet, which makes the process a lot easier. It is recommend that you print the list out and make sure that your fridge and pantry is fully stocked with ONLY these items. Experiment with different recipes in order to make your meals fun and exciting. Clear your kitchen from any form of temptation.

Lean meat

Beef tenderloin

Filet mignon

Buffalo

Extra-lean ham

Extra-lean Kosher beef hot dogs

Lean center-cut pork chops

Lean slices of roast beef

Pork tenderloin, pork loin roast

Reduced-fat bacon

Soy bacon

Steak: flank

Sirloin

London broil

Veal chops

Veal scaloppini

Venison

Poultry

Chicken

Chicken liver

Cornish hen

Fat-free turkey and chicken sausages

Low fat deli slices of chicken or turkey

Ostrich steak

Quail

Turkey

Wild duck

Reduced-fat bacon

Soy bacon

Steak: flank

Sirloin

London broil

Veal chops

Veal scaloppini

Venison

Fish

Arctic char

Catfish

Cod

Flounder

Grouper

Haddock

Halibut and smoked halibut

Herring

Mackerel

Mahi Mahi

Monkfish

Orange roughy

Perch

Red snapper

Salmon or smoked salmon

Sardines, fresh or canned in water

Sea bass

Shark

Sole

Surimi

Swordfish

Tilapia

Trout

Tuna, fresh or canned in water

Shellfish

Clams
Crab
Crawfish, crayfish
Lobster
Mussels

Octopus
Oysters
Scallops
Shrimp
Squid

Vegetarian Proteins

Seitan
Soy foods and veggie burgers
Tempeh
Tofu

Fat-free dairy products

Fat-free cottage cheese
Fat-free cream cheese
Fat-free milk

Fat-free plain Greek style yogurt
Fat-free ricotta
Fat-free sour cream

Eggs

Chicken
Quail
Duck

Vegetables

Artichoke
Asparagus
Bean sprouts
Beetroot (in moderation, as they are starchy)
Broccoli
Brussels sprouts
Cabbage
Carrots (in moderation, as they are starchy)
Cauliflower
Celery
Cucumber
Eggplant
Endive
Fennel
Green beans
Kale
Lettuce
Mushrooms
Onion
Okra
Palm hearts
Peppers
Pumpkin
Radish
Rhubarb
Spaghetti squash
Spinach
Squash
Tomatoes
Turnip
Watercress
Zucchini

CHAPTER 7

Recipe Ideas

M eals on the Dukan Diet do not have to be boring and bland. Have fun in the kitchen, and find ways to make all your meals delicious. *Here are some great recipe ideas:*

Attack Phase

The secret to the Attack Phase is to add flavor to your meals through herbs, spices and a bit of creativity. You can still create delicious and versatile meals in this phase with just a few clever tweaks. This is important because you want to have an element of ease throughout this stage. Also, don't get too disheartened, and remember that this stage is the shortest out of all four, and you won't be here for long. However, it is an important stage where you WILL lose the most weight, so stick it out! We've put together a few simple yet tasty recipes for you to enjoy.

Spicy Chicken Omelet – An omelet is a great way of jazzing things up a bit in the Attack Phase, which can sometimes get quite boring after a while. Let's take a look at how you can create a spicy omelet to enjoy:

Ingredients:

2 eggs (and 1 egg white if you want a bigger omelet)
Half a de-seeded green chili, chopped up finely
Half an onion
½ tsp of dried oregano or thyme

½ tsp of paprika
Salt and pepper
Chicken breast, shredded

Method:

1. Crack the eggs open into a bowl and mix with the salt and pepper.
2. Add the rest of the ingredients and whisk further.

3. Pour the mixture into a non-stick pan which you have slightly greased with olive oil and heat up to medium.
4. Flip both sides until lightly golden. Add chicken pieces and fold in half.

Turkey Burger – Yes, you can still enjoy burgers in the Attack Phase. Sure, they might not have bread rolls or fries on the side but that doesn't mean they can't be delicious. Also you can make a lot of these and then freeze them to eat throughout the week.

Ingredients:

8oz (250g) of lean ground turkey (if you'd prefer another type of ground meat, such as beef or chicken, that is fine too)
Half an onion, diced finely

1 egg
1/2 tsp of paprika
½ tsp coriander or mixed herbs
Salt and pepper

Method:

1. Mix the ground meat and the chopped onion together with the herbs. Add salt and pepper and mix together.
2. Add the egg and continue to mix.
3. Divide the mixture in two to create two burger patties (or more if you are going to double or triple the ingredients).
4. Fry one side then the other until it is cooked to your liking.

Spicy Lemon Roast Chicken – Your chicken recipes don't have to be bland just because you are in the Attack Phase. Spice things up!

Ingredients:

Whole free-range chicken
6 slices of lemon

2 tbsps of tandoori spice mix, or if you want to make your own, just combine 1 tsp ground ginger, 1 tsp ground cumin, 1 tsp ground coriander, 1 tsp paprika, 1 tsp turmeric, 1 tsp salt and 1 tsp cayenne pepper

Method:

1. Preheat oven to 350° F (180° Celsius).
2. Place the chicken in a roasting tin and rub some of the tandoori spice under the layer of skin. Place 3 slices of lemon under the skin, too. Turn the chicken over and repeat the process.

3. Place the roasting tin in the oven and cook for around one and a half hours to two hours. Take the chicken out after about 70 minutes to see how the cooking process is going and to determine how much longer you have to cook it.
4. Remove the chicken from the oven, take off the skin and enjoy.

Turkey Meatballs – Let's face it, the most exciting thing about spaghetti and meatballs is not the pasta but the meat. So skip the spaghetti, and enjoy more meatballs.

Ingredients:

16 oz (500g) ground turkey (or any other ground meat that you like)
1 egg
¼ cup of fat free cottage cheese
1 tbsp mustard (optional)
½ tsp dried parsley

½ tsp dried oregano
2 garlic cloves
1 onion
4 tbsps oat bran
Olive oil spray

Method:

1. Preheat oven to 350° F (180° Celsius).
2. Finely dice the onion and garlic and fry for five minutes.
3. Place all the ingredients into a bowl and mix well.
4. Spray a baking tray with a bit of olive oil spray.
5. Roll the mixture into meatballs in any size you want and place them in a baking tray. Try to keep a bit of space between each one.
6. Bake in the oven for 40 minutes, making sure you turn them halfway through.
7. Enjoy.

Cruise Phase

The Cruise Phase is an exciting change from the Attack Phase, and you'll be surprised at how happy you are to see vegetables. Where pizza and chocolate might have excited you before, you'll now be pleasantly surprised at how much joy a simple vegetable can bring. Vegetables make a great addition to any meal, making them taste better as well as allowing you to stay fuller for longer.

Ground Meat Stuffed Peppers – This delicious meal is perfect for the cruise phase, incorporating both protein and vegetables into one delicious meal.

Ingredients:

4 red peppers
300g of lean ground beef (or whatever ground meat you prefer)
1 egg

4 tbsps of oat bran
2 cloves of garlic
1 tsp of paprika
Salt and pepper

Method:

1. Preheat oven to 350° F (180° Celsius).
2. Cut the peppers in half, and remove any seeds or white flesh.
3. Place the peppers on a roasting tin which has been lined with greaseproof paper, and cook for about 20 minutes or until you see them start to soften.
4. While these are cooking, you can prepare the stuffing by mixing all the left over ingredients together and mixing them well.
5. When the peppers are ready, take them out and fill with the ground beef mixture.
6. Bake in the oven for 30 minutes until the meat is cooked through.
7. Enjoy.

Beef Stew – This makes a great change from the Attack Phase where you were allowed beef but making a beef stew was not possible. So here is a great recipe for you to enjoy in the Cruise Phase:

Ingredients:

8oz (250g) of lean beef, cut in cubes
2 medium carrots, diced
2 tbsps of corn flour
8oz (250g) shallots, cut into pieces
Sliced mushrooms

2 cups (470 ml) of low sodium beef stock
1 tsp of dried thyme
1 tsp of dried rosemary
1 butternut cut into cubes
Salt and pepper

Method:

1. Preheat oven to 350° F (180° Celsius)
2. Coat the beef in the corn flour and then in a pan fry in a bit of oil until lightly seared.
3. Transfer the beef to a casserole dish and add all the other ingredients including the beef stock. Make sure the meat and vegetables are just covered in the liquid.

4. Put a lid on the casserole dish and cook in the oven for two hours or until the meat is tender and cooked through.
5. If you are used to added rice or pasta to your stew, then it is optional to add Shirataki noodles.

Chili con Dukan – The best part about the Dukan Diet is that you can take recipes that you know and love and change them so that they are still allowed in your new eating plan. One of the most loved and comforting meals that people enjoy is Chili con Carne. So here is a revamped version, which we call Chili Con Dukan.

Ingredients:

16oz (500g) ground beef or ground turkey

2 cans of chopped tomatoes

8oz (250g) mushrooms

1 red onion

1 tbsp olive oil

4 tbsps chili powder

2 ½ tsps ground coriander

2 ½ tsps ground cumin

1 ½ tsps garlic powder

1 tsp dried oregano

½ tsp cayenne pepper

½ cup (125ml) boiling water

4 tbsps low fat yogurt (unflavored)

Salt and pepper

Method:

1. Preheat oven to 350° F (180° Celsius).
2. Mix all the ingredients together except for the yogurt.
3. Place the mix into an ovenproof casserole dish and cover with a lid.
4. Place in the oven and cook for 90 minutes, stirring a few times throughout that time.
5. Once done, drizzle the yogurt on top.
6. Enjoy.

Chicken Salad – Salads are great to include into your diet because they can be eaten for lunch or dinner and can be changed every day into something different. On winter days you can even add warm vegetables to the salad, and on summer days you can create a cool and refreshing salad.

Ingredients:

7oz (200g) of shredded chicken

Cucumber, sliced and diced

2 small tomatoes, diced

Slices of red and green pepper

1 carrot, grated

Herbs

Lettuce

Lemon juice

Olive oil

Low-fat plain yogurt

Salt and pepper

Method:

1. Fry the chicken in a bit of olive oil until cooked.
2. Mix all the ingredients together, adding the chicken, lemon juice, a drop of olive oil and salt and pepper at the end.
3. Drizzle yogurt over the top.

Consolidation and Stabilization Phase

Mushroom muffins – This is a great recipe to which you can add many other ingredients to your liking. You can therefore make this each week and have it taste completely different. Here is a simple mushroom muffin idea as your base, however feel free to change it up by adding bacon or other protein to the mix. This is a great recipe to make at the start of the week so you'll have some breakfast or lunches on the go.

Ingredients:

1 tbsp of unsalted butter

1 onion, diced

Herbs, such as dried thyme

8oz (250g) mushrooms, sliced

4oz (110g) reduced fat Swiss cheese

4 whole eggs and 4 egg whites

2 tbsps skim milk

Salt and pepper

Method:

1. Preheat oven to 350° F (180° Celsius)
2. Sauce the onions in butter until they are golden brown.
3. Sauce the mushrooms in some butter with salt and pepper until they are soft and cooked to your liking.
4. Mix the mushroom and onions together and add the thyme.
5. Whisk the whole eggs and egg whites with milk, salt, pepper and cheese.
6. Add to the mushroom and onion mix.

7. Spoon the mixture into your muffin tins and bake for about 15 minutes or until the tops are golden.

Shepherd's Pie – One of the best ways to create Dukan meals is to take foods that you normally eat and give them a Dukan twist. Shepherd's Pie is a fantastic and delicious example of this:

Ingredients:

1 onion

16oz (400g) ground lamb or beef

Herbs

50 oz (1400g) can of chopped tomatoes

¼ cup (50ml) water

7oz (200g) butternut, chopped into cubes

8 ½oz (250g) cauliflower, chopped

Salt and pepper

Cheese (optional)

Method:

1. Preheat oven to 350° F (180° Celsius).
2. Fry the ground meat with onion and a little bit of olive oil.
3. When it's almost finished cooking add the herbs, the can of chopped tomatoes and the water.
4. Bring to the boil, then simmer for twenty minutes.
5. While this is cooking, cook the butternut and cauliflower in a steamer or in a bowl of boiling water until soft and tender.
6. When done drain the water and mash them up.
7. Pour the ground meat mixture into an ovenproof dish and top with the butternut and cauliflower mixture.
8. Bake for 15 minutes.
9. Sprinkle the cheese on top.

Conclusion

Thank you again for downloading this book!

Congratulations on taking the first step towards a healthier lifestyle. The Dukan Diet has proven methods to help you get to the weight that you have always wanted and to finally find happiness in yourself. It teaches you a lot about nutrition and the importance of a happy lifestyle through positive food choices. Remember to be kind to yourself through this process and to allow yourself to go through the phases at your own pace. You are unique and every person will move through the phases differently. Mostly, get excited, because your life is about to change for the better.

The best part about this diet is that you can take it one step at a time until eventually you look back and see how far you have come. Also, because the first phase is the part that produces the biggest weight loss, you will be motivated immediately to continue with the plan. There is a reason that so many people lose weight on this diet and a reason that they keep it off. This is not just a fad diet, but one that has been carefully designed to suit all body types. You'll be surprised at how much weight you will lose and how good you will feel throughout the process. Soon, this will become a way of life.

Best of luck on this exciting journey!

Finally, if you enjoyed this book, then I'd like to ask you for a favor, would you be kind enough to leave a review for this book on Amazon? It'd be greatly appreciated!

Be sure to check out our website at www.thetotalevolution.com for more information.

Thank you!

Our Other Books

Below you'll find some of our other books that are popular on Amazon.com and the international sites.

Master Cleanse: How To Do A Natural Detox The Right Way And Lose Weight Fast

Mayo Clinic Diet: A Proven Diet Plan For Lifelong Weight Loss

Glycemic Index Diet: A Proven Diet Plan For Weight Loss and Healthy Eating With No Calorie Counting

Clean Eating Diet: A 10 Day Diet Plan To Eat Clean, Lose Weight And Supercharge Your Body

Wheat Belly: The Anti-Diet - A Guide To Gluten Free Eating And A Slimmer Belly

IIFYM: Flexible Dieting - Sculpt The Perfect Body While Eating The Foods You Love

Mediterranean Diet: 101 Ultimate Mediterranean Diet Recipes To Fast Track Your Weight Loss & Help Prevent Disease

Acid Reflux Diet: A Beginner's Guide To Natural Cures And Recipes For Acid Reflux, GERD And Heartburn

Hypothyroidism Diet: Natural Remedies & Foods To Boost Your Energy & Jump Start Your Weight Loss

It Starts With Food: A 30 Day Diet Plan To Reset Your Body, Lose Weight And Become A Healthier You

Made in the USA
Las Vegas, NV
15 January 2021

15921929R00025